The PTSD Project

Turn Pain To Power

Reverend Mike Wanner

Table of Contents

Table of Contents _____ 3
Dedication _____ 4
Acknowledgements _____ 5
Chapter 1 - Understanding A Need _____ 7
Chapter 2 - The Process _____ 9
Chapter 3 - Your Story _____ 11
Chapter 4 - What You Should Include In Your Story _____ 18
Chapter 5 - Where You Are _____ 20
Chapter 6 - Elimination of Limitations _____ 22
Chapter 7 - Write A New Story _____ 25
Chapter 9 - Emotional Healing Through Spiritual Energy _____ 28
Chapter 10 - Session & Training Options _____ 29
Chapter 11 - Connections _____ 31
ReverendMikeWanner.com Resources List _____ 32
Private Channeling _____ 35
Rev. Mike Wanner _____ 37

Copyright Reverend Mike Wanner, 2014

Dedication

This book is dedicated to all those who have served to defend the United States of America and their families who have served also, by missing them during their service and some forever. These valiant citizens have given freely in the pursuit of the noble goals specified in the Declaration of Independence and the Constitution of The United States and all the amendments thereto.

I give special recognition to those who have been killed in the service of our country. The citizens now and future citizens of the United States of America will be forever in their debt. May all who have served and their families be blessed in the now and the forever AND SO IT IS!

Special recognition goes also to those injured in the service of our country. The United States of America will be forever in their debt. The injured warriors of our nation have performed well a duty and this writing is offered to help mitigate some of the emotional turmoil that may still reside within those valiant ones. May each of them and their families be blessed in all ways AND SO IT IS!

It is the intent of this work to help Veterans to reclaim their power after their military service is complete.

May All who Read this book be Blessed AND SO IT IS!

Reverend Mike Wanner

Acknowledgements

I would like to acknowledge the support of the following beings:

Ceil Nuyianes is an Earth Angel who started as a student of mine in Reiki and developed into a friend whose book industry expertise helped guide me in many ways.

Mary E Jay who has been an inspiration.

Nancy Russell who was my Integrated Energy Therapy Master Instructor who introduced me to Angel Ariel and the methodology of Heartlinking with the Angels to facilitate the clearing of stuffed emotions and cellular memory.

Stevan Thayer who was my Integrated Energy Therapy Master Instructor Trainer who taught me how to teach others - How to Heal with The Energy of Angels.

My Reiki Masters Rita Hildenbrandt, Hannelore Goodwin, Gary Jirauch, Tom Rigler, Patrick Zigler, Hiroshi Doi, Chiyoko Yamaguchi, Tadao Yamaguchi and especially the founder of Komyo Kai Reiki Reverend Hyakuten Inamoto.

Reverend Ethel Lomardi who taught me the healing power of viewing people as pure light.

Archangels Michael - the Protector, Gabriel - the Communicator, Raphael - the Healer and the legions of Angels that help the healing process for all.

Chapter 1 - Understanding A Need

The Greatest Physician is God Almighty who may be accessed by all always but may not be part of a lot of treatment protocols. The separation of science and spirituality creates a crevice of misunderstanding that is difficult to bridge.

The health care system specialty standards evolve from the experiences of many situations and the consensus of the many practitioners. Please understand that agreement can be hard to attain when the experiences in individual cases can vary widely.

A traditional holistic model which is more whole than traditional care talks about Body, Mind and Spirit and that is definitely a more realistic approach than those that focus only on the body. I feel very definitely that the key to healing has four parts.

My book *Four Parts to Healing* explains that we need four levels of support in order to heal. We need physical support, emotional support, mental support, and spiritual support.

This book will focus on options for applying emotional support to Post Traumatic Stress Disorder - PTSD. This book is not intended to replace any professional services that may be offered and appropriate for any PTSD conditions.

This book is intended to simply provide comfort and understanding so that a more peaceful path to healing may be followed. Notice what all is available for your care and then notice also the array of spiritual options here and elsewhere that can bring you peace and comfort in the process of your healing.

Chapter 2 - The Process

The first thing to appreciate is that traditional protocols have value and are awesome in many ways. The objectivity of traditional diagnostic evaluation allows for specificity in focus and is priceless in your care.

The area that needs attention in many folks is the energetic alignment of the individuals. There is great emotional understanding and power that can be brought to the alignment of your energy.

Turning pain in to power can ease the journey of one that is being challenged. Thoughts amplify the comprehension of the intensity of pain and can contribute intensity to that pain.

What you focus on increases in your life so be careful what you focus on. The Law of Attraction amplifies the power of your focus.

That Law does not only focus on bringing you what you want but also brings you exactly what you don't want when you focus on it. Be careful what you focus on.

Many people that I tell this to look at me and say –Duh! These people act like it is simple and then they just miss the point.

Have you ever listened to a lot of old people talking about their diseases. They own their diseases and program themselves for their future discomfort when certain triggers happen. Please don't do that.

I invite you to focus only on good that you would like to have in your life, create that view of reality and then manifest that good to your absolute delight. Please remember that what you focus on increases in your life so focus on only what you want.

Release thoughts that no longer serve you and choose to think positively about all things. You will manifest things in your life that never before seemed possible.

Chapter 3 - Your Story

When you speak, you are also listening to what you say and then you believe what you say. So if you say the wrong thing about yourself, you create a story and part of your life that is unreal.

You can change your story at any time so I encourage you to start the process of understanding by answering a few things about your PTSD episodes.

When do they occur?_____

Is there a certain something that triggers them?_____

Are you doing a certain thing immediately prior to an episode?_____

Do you journal your episodes?_____

Are you willing to journal your episodes?_____

Are you willing to sit and write your whole Story?____

Do you believe that God can help you if you will open to connect? _____

Will you schedule time in each week to start your story journal now? _____

Why Your Story Is Important

A house is built on a foundation and if the foundation is a mess then so will be the rest of the house. Your life is built on your foundation so you need to be sure it receives the support it needs from time to time.

It is difficult to objectively view your foundational story when you are actively inside it. There is great value in stopping the clock metaphorically and recording where you are to the best of your ability.

Your story now does not limit you in any way. It is like intersection signs that show you where you are. Staying at your story intersection can limit you so I do not recommend it.

If you get stuck in now and have no target destination, you can't go where you have not decided to go. Unfortunately, many people arrive at a story intersection and get stuck there for a considerable time.

Getting stuck is not limited to any particular group of people. Movie Stars are as vulnerable as military people, business executives, teachers and housewives.

Imagine that all kinds of people in your community have PTSD from different sources and you may never know their story. Know that each of them may be able to say something that can help you. Listen.

Know also that you can reciprocate by paying attention to their needs so that you can at least offer them your understanding which may be life-saving. It may be difficult for you to imagine but one word of encouragement at a pivotal time can save a life.

Buddy Up

If you read a buddy's foundational story journal, you could quickly see that there is a clear path in which to move. Since you are not involved, it is easier for you to see issues easier than the writer.

If that same buddy reads your journal, s/he can objectively see the next little step that you need to take. So then both you and your buddy start moving down the highway of life in route to your optimized destination.

Why the Questions?

So let' consider the why of the questions asked above:

1. When do your PTSD episodes occur?

It is important to understand the timing of your episodes as it is a component that can frame some patterns that might be misunderstood without that variant.

2. Is there a certain something that triggers your episodes?

If an episode is always preceded by a predictable trigger, control of the triggering events can be a tool to control the episodes. Acknowledgement of your triggers can be comforting to you as you know what to avoid so that you are triggered less often.

3. Are you doing a certain thing immediately prior to an episode?

What you are doing prior to an episode that is not perceived as a trigger may also be a path to a trigger situation which while it is not an immediate cause can be a preparatory situation that sets the stage for an episode which can then be triggered by any number of otherwise inconsequential things.

3. Do you journal your episodes?

Journaling your episodes is a great tool to help yourself or any practitioner that you are working with at the time. Professional time is very expensive but your notes can cut short the process of information gathering that they need to attain a baseline for where you are at the starting point.

4. Are you willing to journal your episodes?

Knowing you should and actually doing journaling are two entirely different things. If you are serious about healing, begin to do the journaling as it is a taking charge type of decision that says to yourself that you are serious about healing and you will take the initiative to do whatever it takes to heal.

5. Are you willing to sit and write your whole Story?

Being willing to write your story is the beginning point of a Journey of self- discovery. This is not a time to be careful about hiding the truth from your-self.

If you are concerned about somebody finding and reading your story then take precautions to protect it wherever it physically is or password protect it if it is on your computer. A good way to satisfy yourself that it is safe is to put somebody else's name on it. Billy Smith's Journal or Gladys Jones 's journal is not yours and you can deny it if it is found accidentally.

6. Do you believe that God can help you if you will open to connect?

God can help you if you invite God. Some folks have reservations about God and can block the good that God offers.

You beliefs are a big part of your healing and the degree of your doubt can knock you out. Don't play games. You are too important.

Chapter 4 - What You Should Include In Your Story

Your story should be a detailed account of where you came from and what the situation is now. Include cultural references to your family ancestry, education, family business, religion, chronic family illnesses, marital status, etc.

As you review the list of items below, try to be aware of the emotions that come up and record them. Especially include feelings of heartache, betrayal, anger, fear and rage.

Consider if the following influence your old story:

Race

Age

Living Locations

Education

Family culture

Family Business

Religious Upbringing

Family Illnesses

Marital Status

Military Service

Identified Traumas/Crimes

Medical History with Ages

Drug Dependency – Prescription

Drug Dependency – Street Drugs

Smoking

Alcohol Use

Family Crisis – Immediate Family

Family Crisis – Extended Family

Get to Work on Your Story –

Step one - Get a notebook or start a computer page

Step Two - Answer the questions in Chapter 3

Step Three - Consider the influences in this chapter above.

Step Four – Write out the truth of where you are including all the problems, opportunities, hurdles, challenges and your disappointments. Finish with a resolution of what three things you would like to change and which one of them is first.

Chapter 5 - Where You Are

You have been dealt a hand in life. If you are not Royalty, You may not like it.

If you don't like it, Get real and Change the Deal. Drop the "'T" off "I can't" and make it "I can"

It's your life, you are in charge and you are the dealer. Shuffle the cards and begin to play within your own rules.

But how you say – "Can I change things?" That's simple: You change things by thinking about them differently.

Start walking on the path to Release. Acknowledge how you feel. Undo the lock that stress has on you by owning your feelings and asking for help. Who do you ask?

You may wish to say "God Help Me change."

You may not. Some people understand about God, whoever and whatever you believe God to be, and others just don't.

I believe that you can change things a lot easier with God's help but that is not for everyone so I cover many techniques. You always have a choice in life even when it feels that you do not.

Chapter 6 - Elimination of Limitations

Here is the technique for the Elimination of Limitations.

MAKE A LIST OF YOUR "I CANT'S" Spend some time on it. Make sure you have them all.

Grade each with a priority code. Grade them A, B, C, D. A will equal the worst of the worst or you could say your best of the "I cant's" or you could say the things you absolutely can't do. Put them down on the list.

B will equal the next level of difficulty.

C will equal the next level of difficulty.

D will equal the least difficult things that you can't do.

Next, prioritize them in descending order from 10 (the worst) to 1 (the least) within their alphabetical grade. You would have A10 to A1, B10 to B1, C10 to C1, D10 to -D1. Yes you can have more that one of each but if you have a lot of one then you will need to further prioritize with sub-lists.

Print or write out the list in descending priority order.

Now that you have done all that work, give yourself a pat on the back because you are working at taking charge of your life and there are few more noble tasks. You are polishing the diamond that you are.

You are creating sparkle in your life, your family and your community. You are on your way to your power. Now get to work on this list.

Start with the Least D1. Get a pen or pencil (red if you have it) and take your D1 and make an x over the "'T" or get an eraser (Liquid or rubber) and remove the "'T". Make the remaining "I can" your affirmation for 3 days at least or as many as 21. "I can _____. " Say it at least three times a day, preferably a lot more. Take some action (one step minimum each day) towards the fulfillment of D1. Notice how it feels to do that.

Next, start with the worst. Get a pen or pencil (red if you have it) and take your A10 and make a red x over the "'T" or get an eraser (liquid or rubber) and remove the "'T". Make the remaining "I can" your affirmation for 3 days at least or as many as 21. "I can _____. " Say it at least 3 times a day, preferably a lot more. Take some action (one step minimum each day) towards the fulfillment of A10. Notice how it feels to do that.

Take your next lowest and then your next highest. Etc.

WOW! After all that work, it is time to reward yourself. Remember to be gentle with yourself as you work to polish the diamond that you are.

Chapter 7 - Write A New Story

You can create for yourself a story of how you would like your life to be. Take every item from above and write the new story with your clearing and eliminations fully implemented.

Tell the tale of your power and manifestations as completely as you can envision. Put down every detail as vibrantly as you can.

You have done a lot if you are following my instructions. You have found out where you are and formed new thought patterns as to what you can do.

You have started the process of changing your thinking to align with a new reality that would be much more to your liking. You have created a vision of the path that will take you to the destination.

Congratulations. You have done a lot and your new story can serve you well and open many doors for you with the traditional care system. Take your notes with you and/OR-

Chapter 8 - Choose To Participate In This Project

The reality behind this project is that I am laying out criteria to help provide a foundation for those afflicted with PTSD so they can find some folks that can help. There are people out there that want to help but there does not seem to be a track in which they can run.

Hopefully my last statement is inaccurate and many are receiving all the help they need now. I doubt that.

Just the other day at the VA hospital, I encountered a fellow veteran who was going off on a clerk. He said nothing helps. Just a little understanding settled him right down and the clerk and the veteran and I also breathed a sigh of relief.

"The drugs wear off and I can't sleep and because of that I have no patience", he said. I looked in to his eyes and saw terror and he looked into mine and saw understanding.

He was shortly called for his appointment and he thanked me and I thanked him. It is so gratifying to me when I know that the one I am talking to understands that I understand.

Trying to understand has been a calling of my life. This work is an effort to understand even more.

The government could set aside billions to tackle this problem or perhaps we can create an environment of caring that has beneficial results with some coordination of efforts.

I am not an expert about PTSD and am very open to collaboration with anyone out there who has programs or efforts that can interact with what I am suggesting.

I am hopeful that the concepts covered in my book "Tea For Veterans: Welcome One Home" are already helping to establish a support net for returning veterans. That book and five others are offered free periodically on Kindle. You can add your name to the notification list as
http://VeteransHealing.withRevMike.com

Chapter 9 - Emotional Healing Through Spiritual Energy

There are spiritual healing modalities that can be applied in person or at a distance. Think of the practitioner as a sender of energy and the client as a receiver of energy.

I propose and will focus my comments on two modalities that are spiritual energy techniques that use spiritual energy to support clients. More information on these techniques can easily be found on the internet.

The modalities that I would like to suggest are Reiki and Integrated Energy Therapy®. I use both modalities together in my sessions and use more Reiki when the biggest need is physical and more Integrated Energy Therapy® when the biggest need is emotional.

You may find more of one modality in your neighborhood so follow your heart and wisdom. Prayers for guidance can be very fruitful. Both modalities are effective for physical and emotional and mental and spiritual support.

Chapter 10 - Session & Training Options

Thankfully there are many folks that do healing energy work on a Pro Bono basis and this is a great place to start your journey to additional acceleration for your PTSD recovery. If you are able to connect with a sender who works Pro Bono, then you are indeed fortunate.

The problem becomes about quantity of energy needed. Volunteers are willing to give and many give a lot according to their availability and personal energy. Spend some time searching for one that might help you.

There are also professional energy practitioners who are well worth their fees. Of course, the fact that they are professionals means that they are likely to have honed their skills to a high level of proficiency and perhaps that level may help you over trouble spots whether you can stay with them or not.

Consider your needs but also consider that there are also teachers who can teach you to do the modalities for yourself and others. The teachers also are well worth their fees.

I have created the cheapest option that I can figure as a new modality that is little known. I call it Crisis Reiki and at times I have called it Crisis? Reiki! Baby? Reiki!. A complete explanation of the idea is available at http://www.CrisisReiki.com.

The idea for anyone with a Crisis or who is preparing to have a baby is to choose to try a treatment, a Reiki 1 class or an abbreviated training that I outline on the website.

The idea is simply that some Reiki is better than no Reiki and someone in crisis with little resources may benefit from a single attunement with an abbreviated class.

Perhaps, the right series of resources for you might involve free and paid resources that can carry you long enough to learn how to do energy healing for yourself and others.

Chapter 11 - Connections

The first paperback book that I released was called *Angel Raphael Speaks Volume One.* The same messages contained in that book and ninety more are on the website http://www.AngelRaphaelSpeaks.com. Angel Raphael is the Angel of Healing and I invite you to pray to him for guidance.

On that website, I have added a tab called Veterans and you can leave a comment/reply there of what your needs might be and you can leave a request to give or receive spiritual energy. I offer it as a site where you might connect with someone who can help you.

That page is not like ordering from a catalog but it is more like a forum opportunity where you put your needs out and look to see what may be offered by others. You would be wise to continue your search on the internet. Forums are unpredictable.

One of the strongest things that you can do for yourself is to pray for others. Selflessness is Godly.

May all who read this be blessed, AND SO IT IS!

ReverendMikeWanner.com Resources List

Distant Healing Sessions –

Physical Healing
http://LetMeHelpYouHeal.withMike.com

Angel Healing
http://AngelHealing.withmike.com/

Books by Rev. Mike at www.Amazon.com–

Veterans Healing Six Pack:
1. *Trauma Healing options for VA Hospitals: Help for Veterans to Own Their Healing and their future.*
2. *Trauma Healing Action Steps for Veterans: Help to Start Healing*
3. *Trauma Healing Action Steps for Veterans: Empowerment*
4. *Trauma Healing Action Steps for Veterans: Forgiveness*
5. *Trauma Healing Action Steps for Veterans: Thought Freedom*
6. *Tea For Veterans: Welcome One Home*

Angel Raphael Speaks Volume One: Take Courage! God Has Healing in Store for You

Angel Raphael Speaks Volume Two: Take Courage! God Has Healing in Store for You

Reiki Journaling from Japan

Reiki Is Alive: God's Great Gift

Four Parts to Healing

Distant Healing: We Are All Connected

Stress Release Energy Work: How To Cope

Does Reiki Love Heal Cancer?

Group Consciousness

Free Resources

Learn to dump fear at
http://TheGreatAmericanFearDump.withMike.com

Spiritually Prepare for Surgery
http://PrepareForSurgery.withRevMike.com

Angel Scribe messages at
http://www.SpiritualComfortCare.com

Law of Attraction Expert column at
http://www.ReverendMikeWanner.com

Stress Release at
http://www.StressReleaseCoach.com

    Angel Raphael Speaks through Rev. Mike Wanner. I have channeled multiple message sets and they all have to be polished to smooth out my errors and negotiate some words that may be too easily misunderstood. Grammar is not polished as it is too easy to miss the subtlety of the energy flow. To find out the availability of messages and latest updates go to http://www.spiritualcomfortcare.com/angel-raphael-speaks/

Also "Tell Mike your concerns – If he and I agree there is a broader need, messages may follow. Citizens of all nations invited as long as your write in English. Do not expect him to answer as he is very busy already listening to us." E-mail Mike at mikewann@voicenet.com.

    May All Who Read This Be Blessed Reverend Mike Wanner

Join the Veterans Healing FREE Kindle Book Notification List at http://VeteransHealing.withRevMike.com

Private Channeling

Angel Raphael Speaks is a series of free messages that are channeled through Reverend Mike Wanner for the Highest good and Highest Healing of all concerned.

Many questions arise about Reverend Mike doing private channeling and he does help with that at his site
http://AngelHealing.withMike.com

Reverend Mike is available world-wide as a psychic channel, emotional release facilitator, spiritual energy practitioner & teacher, and public speaker. He looks forward to meeting you soon!

Email - mikewann@voicenet.com 215-342-1270
http://AngelHealing.withMike.com

PRIVATE SPIRITUAL READINGS/channelings or Spiritual Healing Sessions: Telephone or in person

Rev. Mike is available for private, one-on-one intuitive sessions with you, his Guide Family, and your Guides. He helps by offering clarity on emotional situations about your life, your purpose, your spirituality, and the release of stuffed emotions and cellular memory.

Connect to the love of your Guides today!

Contact Rev. Mike for an appointment.

Click on this link to go to the page –
http://AngelHealing.withMike.com

Sessions available:

Spiritual Readings
Angel Channeling
Distant Reiki Healing
Distant Clearing of Stuffed Emotions
Distant Clearing of Cellular Memory
Distant Clearing of Energy Blockages
Distant Clearing of the Chakras
Mastermind dowsing responses to yes/no direction finding questions.
Customized needs

Rev. Mike is a facilitator of healing. He brings you and the Divine together so that you can align with the Divine and have a great time and a great life. All healing is between you and God, as it should be. Go ahead and start without Rev. Mike. Visit his prayer site http://www.Create-A-Prayer.com. Take the first step NOW.

Rev. Mike Wanner

Rev. Mike Wanner started his metaphysical and ministerial studies with Reiki in 1993 and has studied seven styles of Reiki in the U.S., Japan, Canada, Denmark and Australia. He is certified to teach. He became certified to teach Integrated Energy Therapy in 1999 and co-taught the first IET class of the new Millennium. Mike began dowsing in 2001.

Ordained as a Metaphysical Minister of the International Metaphysical Ministry and an Interfaith Minister of the Circle of Miracles Ministry, Rev. Mike practices and teaches spiritual energy therapies in the Philadelphia Area.

Rev. Mike holds ministerial degrees from the University of Metaphysics and the University of Sedona. He is a Pastoral Care Associate of Aria – Frankford Hospital. He taught at the National Academy of Massage Therapy and Health Sciences.

Rev. Mike was a faculty member of the Medical Mission Sister's Center for Human Integration's School of Integrated Body/Mind Therapies in Fox Chase, Philadelphia, PA for twelve years.

Rev. Mike is licensed by the teaching of Intuitional Metaphysics to practice Spiritual Healing and Scientific Prayer. Mike is also a Prayer therapist.

Rev. Mike was elected in 2007 to the status of "Fellow of the American Institute of Stress."

In 2008, Rev. Mike became a practitioner of Coincidental Recognition as he incorporated the CoRe system in to his spiritual healing practice.

In 2009, Rev. Mike trademarked a new healing process called Quantum Quatro! Subtle Energy System Support®.

In 2011, Rev. Mike joined the outreach program known as the Health Advantage Group.

In 2012. Rev. Mike became a Certified Professional Coach by The Master Coaching Academy and Joined The Personal Empowerment Group .

Prior to his metaphysical, ministerial and coaching studies, Rev. Mike worked for Sears Roebuck and Co. while in High School and after graduation until he joined the U. S. Air Force in 1965. He returned to Sears from Vietnam in 1969 and stayed until 1978. His final Sears assignment was as an efficiency expert in Methods - Operational Research and Development. He volunteered with Burholme Emergency Medical Services from 1969 and is still a Life Member and Board of Directors Member. He started a private ambulance company in 1975 and worked professionally in the field until 2001 when he devoted his full attention to real estate investing, healing and coaching.

www.ReverendMikeWanner.com

CPSIA information can be obtained
at www.ICGtesting.com
Printed in the USA
LVOW12s1527100416
482975LV00026B/597/P

9 781503 211902